Table of Contents

Calories are the units of energy you get from foods and beverages, and when you consume fewer calories than you burn, you achieve a calorie deficit.

The calories you burn or expend each day — also known as calorie expenditure — include the following three components (1Trusted Source):

Resting energy expenditure (REE). REE refers to the calories your body uses at rest for functions that keep you alive, such as breathing and blood circulation.

Thermic effect of food. This involves the calories your body expends digesting, absorbing, and metabolizing food.

Activity energy expenditure. This refers to the calories you expend during sports like exercise and non-exercise related activities, including fidgeting and performing household chores.

If you provide your body fewer calories than it needs to support these three components of calorie expenditure, you put your body into a calorie deficit. Doing so consistently for long periods results in weight loss (1Trusted Source).

Conversely, you will gain weight if you regularly provide your body more calories than it needs to support these functions. This is called a calorie surplus.

BREAKFAST

1. Thai Stir Fried Noodles

Prep Time: 8 Minutes

Cook Time: 10 Minutes

Servings: 2-3

Ingredients

Sauce:

- 200g / 7 oz dried wide rice stick noodles, or 15 oz / 450g fresh wide flat rice noodles
- 2 tsp dark soy sauce
- 1 1/2 tbsp oyster sauce
- 1 tbsp light soy sauce (or all purpose)
- 2 tsp white vinegar (plain white vinegar)
- 2 tsp sugar (any type)

Stir Fry:

- 3 tbsp peanut or vegetable oil , separated
- 2 cloves garlic cloves, very finely chopped

- 1 cup / 150g / 5oz chicken thighs (boneless, skinless), sliced
- 1 large egg
- 4 stems Chinese broccoli

Instructions

1. Chinese Broccoli – trim ends, cut into 7.5cm/3" pieces. Separate leaves from stems. Cut thick stems in half vertically so they're no wider than 0.8cm / 0.3" thick.

2. Noodles – Prepare according to packet directions and drain. Time it so they're cooked just before using – do not leave cooked rice noodles lying around, they break in the wok.

3. Sauce – Mix ingredients until sugar dissolves.

Cooking:

1. Heat oil: Heat 1 tbsp oil in a very large heavy based skillet or wok over high heat.

2. Cook garlic and chicken: Add garlic, cook 15 seconds. Add chicken, cook until it mostly changes from pink to white.

3. Chinese broccoli STEMS: Add Chinese broccoli stems, cook until chicken is almost cooked through.

4. Chinese broccoli LEAVES: Add Chinese broccoli leaves, cook until just wilted.

5. Scramble egg: Push everything to one side, crack egg in and scramble.

6. REMOVE chicken from wok: Remove everything in the wok onto a plate (scrape wok clean).

7. Caramelise noodles: Return wok to stove, heat 2 tbsp oil over high heat until it starts smoking (HOT is key!). Add noodles and Sauce. Toss as few times as possible to disperse Sauce and make edges of noodles caramelise – about 1 to 1 1/2 minutes.

8. Add chicken back in: Quickly add chicken and veg back in, and toss to disperse. Serve immediately!

Prep Time: 5 Minutes

Cook Time: 20 Minutes

Servings: 4

Ingredients

Mushroom Spinach Filling:

- 30g / 2 tbsp unsalted butter
- 200g / 7oz mushrooms , sliced thinly (0.3cm / 1/8")
- 2 cloves garlic , finely minced
- 2 tsp fresh thyme leaves
- 1/4 tsp cooking / salt
- 1/8 tsp black pepper
- 4 cups baby spinach

Baked Eggs:

- 4 large eggs fridge cold
- Pinch salt and pepper
- 1/4 cup thickened cream (heavy cream)
- 4 tbsp parmesan freshly grated
- 1/8 tsp smoked paprika (optional)
- 2 tsp chives, finely chopped (optional)

Instructions

1. Preheat oven to 200°C / 390°F (180°C fan). Lightly oil or butter four ramekins – 300ml / 10oz (1 1/4 cups).

2. Cook mushrooms: Melt butter in a large skillet over medium high heat. Cook mushrooms until starting to go golden on the edges, 3 minutes. Add garlic, thyme, salt and pepper. Cook for further 1 minute until mushrooms and garlic are golden.

3. Wilt spinach: Add spinach and stir for 30 seconds, just until wilted.

4. Fill ramekins: Divide mushroom mixture evenly into the ramekins. Make a slight dent in the middle, crack eggs in (yolk should settle in centre). Sprinkle each egg with pinch of salt and pepper, drizzle with cream, pile on parmesan.

5. Bake: Bake in oven for 12 – 15 minutes until egg whites are just set and yolks are cooked to your liking (I like runny!). Check it at 12 minutes – hotter ovens, lower walled ramekins etc can make them cook faster. Take out of oven slightly undercooked as egg will keep cooking.

6. Paprika: Sprinkle smoked paprika and chives on top, serve immediately with warm bread for dunking!

Prep Time: 15 Minutes

Cook Time: 1hrs 20 Minutes

Servings: 8-12

Ingredients

- 10 eggs
- 3/4 cups cream or milk, full fat best
- 1/2 tsp salt and pepper, each
- 1 1/2 cups shredded cheese (cheddar, tasty, or other of choice)
- 100g/3 oz mushroom, sliced (I used 1 large, optional)
- 100g / 3oz feta , crumbled (optional)

Herb Garlic Roasted Vegetables:

- 2 tbsp olive oil
- 2 garlic cloves, minced
- 3/4 tsp salt
- 1/2 tsp pepper
- 1.5 tsp mixed dried herbs (or uses any of choice)
- 350g / 12oz pumpkin , butternut or sweet potato, 1.7cm / 0.7" cubes

- 2 zucchinis , sliced 1.25 / 0.5" thick rounds
- 1 large red capsicum (bell pepper), sliced

Instructions

Roasted Vegetables:

1. Preheat oven to 220°C/430°F (200°C fan).
2. Toss vegetables on tray with oil, garlic, herbs, salt and pepper. Spread out.
3. Roast 25 minutes, undisturbed (no flipping). Remove and cool for at least 5 minutes before using.

Baked Frittata:

1. Lower oven to 180°C/350°F (160°C fan).
2. Grease & line pan: Spray a 19 x 30cm / 8 x 10" rectangle or 22 cm / 9" square pan lightly with oil, then line with parchment paper with overhang. (Note 3)
3. Egg mixture: Whisk eggs, cream, salt and pepper in a bowl.
4. Assemble: Spread 2/3 of the vegetables in the prepared pan. Pour over egg mixture, sprinkle with cheese, then top with remaining vegetables.

5. Topping: Top with crumbled feta, then mushrooms. Drizzle mushrooms with a touch of olive oil (makes it brown).

6. Bake: Bake 40 minutes until centre is just set.

7. Rest & serve: Rest frittata 5 minutes in the pan. Use paper overhang to lift out of pan, then slice into squares and serve.

8. Serving later: Cool on rack and remove paper from underneath (otherwise base gets soggy). Cut then refrigerate up to 5 days, or freeze. Reheat in microwave.

Prep Time: 15 Minutes

Cook Time: 45 Minutes

Servings: 3

Ingredients

- 1 rack of lamb (6 to 9 bones) your choice Frenched or not
- 1 1/4 tsp salt
- 3/4 tsp black pepper
- 2 tbsp olive oil

Dijon Mustard "Glue":

- 3 tsp egg , lightly whisked
- 3 tbsp Dijon mustard
- 1 tbsp fresh rosemary leaves, finely chopped
- 1 small garlic clove, minced

Garlic Parmesan Crumb:

- 1 cup Panko breadcrumbs
- 2 tbsp parmesan , finely grated
- 1 garlic clove , finely minced (knife, not garlic press)

- 1/4 tsp each salt and pepper
- 2 tbsp fresh rosemary leaves , finely chopped
- 30g / 2 tbsp butter , melted

Creamy White Wine & Mustard Sauce

- 1 cup dry white wine (sauvignon blanc, pinto gris, semillon, or any blend)
- 1 cup chicken stock , low sodium
- 1 cup heavy/thickened cream
- 1 tbsp dijon mustard
- 1/8 tsp each salt and pepper

Instructions

1. Preheat oven to 200°C/390°F (all oven types). Place shelf in the middle of the oven.

Prepare Lamb:

2. Season: Sprinkle lamb rack with salt and pepper.
3. Sear: Heat 1 tbsp oil in a heavy based skillet over high heat. Sear lamb rack all over until nicely browned – including each short end – about 1 1/2 minutes on each side. It will be fully raw inside, but that's OK.

Transfer to plate and let cool for 5 minutes, uncovered.

4. Mustard Spread: Mix dijon, rosemary and garlic in a small bowl. Then add 3 teaspoons of egg, and mix again.

5. Making the crumb: Mix Crumb ingredients EXCEPT butter in a bowl. Then use a fork to stir through butter. Spread on a dinner plate (large enough that fits lamb).

6. Crumbing the lamb: Spread the underside of the rack with mustard mix. Press into breadcrumb mixture, then spread mustard mix over the other side as well as each end. Then press those sides into the breadcrumb mixture.

7. Transfer lamb to rack set on a tray. Surround with parboiled vegetables if using – but don't crowd the lamb.

8. Roast: Frenched racks for 20 minutes, or untrimmed racks for 30 – 35 minutes, or until internal temperature registers 60°C/140°F (for medium rare).

9. Rest meat: Transfer lamb to a cutting board, loosely cover with foil. (If you roasted veg, leave in tray or pan and keep warm in turned off oven).

10. Carve: Rest 5 minutes then slice carefully using your hands to hold the crumb gently in place where you are cutting using a very sharp knife. If your service allows it, it's best to cut 2 or 3 bones together (ie. a double/triple cutlet portion), because the crumb stays on better. Slicing single cutlets is super hard (sadly)!

11. Serve as-is (no sauce), with Creamy White Wine & Mustard Sauce, or Pea Puree.

Creamy White Wine & Mustard Sauce

1. Boil wine and chicken stock together until reduced by 3/4, then whisk in cream and mustard and simmer for 3 – 5 minutes until thickened. The consistency should be a thin pouring sauce. We don't want to coat the lamb too thickly as the sauce flavour will be overpowering.

Prep Time: 15 Minutes

Cook Time: 5 Minutes

Servings: 3-4

Ingredients

- 500g/1 lb asparagus (3 standard Australian bunches)
- 1 1/2 tbsp extra virgin olive oil
- 1/4 tsp each salt and pepper
- 1 garlic clove , finely minced (knife or garlic press)

Optional Finishes:

- 2 tbsp lemon juice
- 2 tbsp parmesan , freshly grated

Instructions

2. Preheat oven to 220°C/430°F (200°C fan).
3. Snap the woody ends off the asparagus – it will naturally break at the right point.
4. Pile onto tray. Drizzle with oil, sprinkle with salt, pepper and garlic. Toss, then spread out on tray.

5. Roast 7 minutes, or until ends have a bit of colour on them and the asparagus is just cooked through. It will take 10 – 12 minutes for very thick ones. Don't let them get wrinkly and sad!

6. Remove from oven.

7. Toss with lemon juice, if using. Pile onto serving platter, grate over optional parmesan. Serve!

Prep Time: 15 Minutes

Cook Time: 15 Minutes

Servings: 4

Ingredients

- 500g/ 1 lb jumbo prawns/shrimp , peeled and deveined
- 3/4 cup dry white wine (sub chicken broth)
- 75g/ 5 tbsp unsalted butter, melted
- 2 tbsp lemon juice
- 3 garlic cloves , minced
- 1/2 tsp salt
- 1/4 tsp pepper

Crunchy Topping:

- 3/4 cup panko breadcrumbs
- 1/4 cup parmesan , finely shredded
- 1/4 tsp salt
- 1.5 tbsp olive oil

GARNISH:

- Finely chopped parsley
- Lemon

Instructions

1. Preheat oven to 220°C/430°F (all oven types).
2. Pour wine and half the butter into 9 x 13" / 22 x 33cm baking pan (if using glass). Place in oven for 10 minutes to reduce.
3. Toss prawns with remaining butter, garlic, lemon juice, salt and pepper. Butter may harden - that's ok.
4. Mix Crunchy Topping ingredients.
5. Remove pan from oven. Add prawns - spread out in single layer, but snug.
6. Top with Crunchy Topping. Bake 12 minutes.
7. Flick to broiler/grill on high, broil for 1 - 2 minutes (max) to brown top a bit more.
8. Sprinkle with parsley. Serve immediately with lemon wedges and crusty bread to mop up the incredible sauce!

Prep Time: 7 Minutes

Cook Time: 5 Minutes

Servings: 1

Ingredients

- 3 egg whites
- 10g/ 1/3 oz pecorino , finely shredded (sub parmesan,)
- 1/2 tsp chives , finely chopped + extra for garnish
- 10g/ 2 tsp unsalted butter
- 1/8 tsp sea salt
- 1 small pinch white pepper

Filling:

- 1 tsp olive oil
- 1/2 cup asparagus , finely sliced on an angle (~2 spears, 25g/1 oz)
- 2 paper-thin slices prosciutto (20g/ 2/3oz)

Instructions

1. Pre-heat oven to 200°C/390°F (180°C fan).

2. First, separate eggs and place whites in a bowl. Reserve yolks for another use.

3. Cook asparagus and prosciutto: Heat olive oil in a 20cm/8" oven-proof, non-stick pan over medium heat. Add asparagus and cook until tender. When almost done, add prosciutto and stir for 30 seconds – just enough to warm through but not crisp. Transfer to a bowl and set aside.

4. Melt butter: Add butter into the same skillet and place over low heat. The butter should melt and be bubbling gently (ie. hot, but not smoking) when the egg whites are ready to pour in.

5. Whisk whites until it's just opaque, fluffy and creamy. Do not take it to "stiff peaks". It should be a consistency so you can draw a figure 8 on the surface and it stays there without sinking. You do not want to be able to do "elf hats" (see in post for photo), that's too stiff. (Whisking time for me: 90 seconds by hand, 30 seconds on Speed 4 electric beater).

6. Add chives, salt and pepper. Whisk a few times just to mix through.

7. Immediately pour egg whites into hot skillet, spread with a spatula to cover surface. Stir for 10 to 12 seconds until the whites start to set on the base.

8. Remove from stove, then lightly tap the pan 5 times on the stove grates or a heat mat to remove bubbles from the base.

9. Sprinkle asparagus, prosciutto and pecorino on half the omelette (the half opposite the handle).

10. Transfer to oven for 2 minutes.

11. Remove from oven. Run rubber spatula around edges and then under the side without the filling, carefully fold omelette in half to cover the filling.

12. Press the omelette's rounded edge against the side of the pan for 30 seconds to seal the edge.

13. Turn out onto plate: Hold a plate at a 45 degree angle. Then flip the omelette out onto the plate so it lands upside down, ie. pan-contact face up (see video for demo).

14. Garnish with chives. Serve immediately!

Prep Time: 17 Minutes

Cook Time: 20 Minutes

Servings: 8-9

Ingredients

- 1/4 cup flour , plain / all purpose
- 1/4 cup cornflour / cornstarch
- 1/4 tsp baking soda (or 3/4 tsp baking powder)
- 1 egg
- 2 tbsp milk (any type)
- 2 cups fresh corn kernels, raw (2 cobs) (canned or frozen also fine)
- 1/2 cup parmesan, finely grated
- 3/4 cup green onions, sliced
- 1/2 cup coriander/cilantro, roughly chopped (sub more green onion)

For Cooking:

- 1/2 cup vegetable oil
- Oil spray

Serving - Choose:

- Avocado sauce
- Sour cream, ketchup (don't judge until you've tried it!)

Instructions

1. Preheat oven to 120°C / 250°F and set a wire rack on a baking tray.
2. Place flour, cornflour and baking soda in a bowl, mix to combine.
3. Add egg and milk, mix until incorporated (batter will be lumpy and thick).
4. Add corn, parmesan, green onions and coriander. Mix until all the corn is evenly coated in batter.
5. Add enough oil into the skillet so it just covers the base. Heat over medium high heat.
6. Spray the underside of a spatula with oil (so batter won't stick when you flatten).
7. Place 1/4 cup batter into skillet (ice cream scooper with lever is handy), then flatten to 1cm thick. Repeat with 2 or 3 more, but don't crowd the skillet.
8. Cook 3 minutes until deep golden and crisp, then flip and cook the other side for 2 – 3 minutes.

9. Transfer to rack and keep warm in oven. Repeat with remaining fritters, using more oil as necessary.

10. Serve with sauce of choice for dunking!

Prep Time: 15 Minutes

Cook Time: 40 Minutes

Servings: 6

Ingredients

Butterscotch Pudding:

- 1/4 cup (50g) dark brown sugar, packed
- 1 1/4 cup (185g) plain flour (all purpose flour)
- 2.5 tsp baking powder
- 100g / 7 tbsp unsalted butter , melted
- 1 egg
- 1/2 cup (125ml) milk (full or low fat)
- 4 tbsp golden syrup

Butterscotch Sauce:

- 3/4 cup (150g) dark brown sugar, packed
- 2 tbsp cornflour / corn starch
- 2 cups (500ml) boiling water

Serving:

- Vanilla ice cream

Instructions

1. Preheat oven to 180°C/350°F (160°C fan).
2. Grease a 6 cup baking dish (1.6L/1.6Q) with butter.
3. Butterscotch Sauce: Whisk sugar and cornflour in bowl. Set aside.
4. Pudding batter: Place sugar, flour and baking powder in a separate bowl. Whisk to combine.
5. Add butter, egg, milk and golden syrup. Whisk until mostly lump free.
6. Scrape into baking dish and smooth surface.
7. Sprinkle Butterscotch Sauce sugar mixture all over surface.
8. Pour boiling water over the surface over the back of a dessert spoon held as close to the batter as you can (to soften the pour so it doesn't break the surface of the batter).
9. Transfer to oven, bake 40 minutes or until skewer inserted into the cake part comes out clean.
10. Cut through pudding to reveal butterscotch sauce underneath.
11. To serve, scoop pudding into a bowl then douse with butterscotch sauce. Top with ice cream!

Prep Time: 10 Minutes

Cook Time: 15 Minutes

Servings: 4

Ingredients

Sausage Patties:

- 1 lb / 500g ground pork (juicier) OR beef (mince)
- 1/2 tsp dried ground sage
- 1/2 tsp dried thyme
- 1 tsp onion powder (or garlic powder)
- 3/4 tsp black pepper
- 3/4 tsp salt
- 1/2 tsp sugar (any)

Muffins:

- 2 tbsp oil
- 4 eggs
- 4 English muffins, cut in half
- 4 slices cheese

Instructions

1. Preheat oven to 130C/275F.
2. Place muffins on a baking tray, cut side up, and top with cheese. (Alternative - melt cheese on sausage patties, see video)

Sausage Patties

1. Mix Sausage Patty ingredients in a bowl - use your hands to mix it real good!
2. Shape into 4 patties (thick ones, or 5 Maccers size patties). Make them slightly larger than the muffins because they will shrink when cooking.
3. Heat oil in a large non stick skillet over high heat. Add patties (in batches if needed). Cook the first side for 2 - 3 minutes or until browned. Flip then cook the other side until browned. (Optional: After flipping, top with cheese, cover with lid to melt).

Egg:

1. Meanwhile, heat another pan over medium high heat with 1 tbsp oil. Spray egg rings with oil and place in the skillet. (Note 4 for other cook methods).
2. Crack egg into the rings. Add around 2 tbsp water into the skillet then cover with a lid. Cook for 1 - 2 minutes

or until egg is cooked to your liking (I like runny yolks).

Assemble:

1. Remove warm muffins from the oven. Top with sausage, then egg, the lid of muffin.
2. Serve and enjoy!

11. Egg Foo Young (Chinese omelette)

Prep Time: 10 Minutes

Cook Time: 15 Minutes

Servings: 4

Ingredients

Sauce :

- 4 tsp cornflour / corn starch
- 1 1/2 tbsp light soy sauce, or all purpose
- 2 tsp Oyster Sauce
- 1 tbsp Chinese Cooking Wine (shaoxing wine) OR Mirin
- 1/2 tsp sesame oil
- 1 cup / 250 ml water
- Dash of white pepper

Omelette:

- 6 eggs
- 2 cups bean sprouts (just eyeball it)
- 4 shallots/green onions, white part only, sliced

- Salt and white pepper

- 2 tbsp vegetable oil

- 1 tsp sesame oil

- 1 garlic clove, finely chopped

One Filling of Choice, below (Prawn or Pork)

- OPTION 1: FOR PRAWN /SHRIMP EGG FOO YOUNG

- 100 – 120g/3.5 – 4 oz chopped raw small prawns/shrimp , peeled and deveined (Note 4)

- OPTION 2: FOR PORK EGG FOO YOUNG :

- 100 – 120g/3.5 – 4 oz ground/mince pork (or chicken, turkey, beef or veal)

- 1/2 tsp EACH soy sauce and Oyster Sauce

- 1/4 tsp sugar

- Dash of sesame oil

Garnish (Optional):

- Sesame seeds, sliced green onion

Instructions

Sauce:

1. Mix cornflour and soy sauce. Then add remaining ingredients.

2. Pour into a saucepan over medium heat. Bring to simmer, stirring constantly. Simmer for 1 minute until sauce thickens to thin syrup consistency. Remove from stove, set aside.

3. MICROWAVE option: Microwave on high for 1 1/2 minutes. Stir very well, microwave for another 1 1/2 minutes until thickened. Mix well again.

Pork Filling:

1. Place pork in a bowl, add remaining ingredients. Use fork to mix through.

Omelette:

2. Whisk eggs in a bowl.

3. Add beansprouts, green onions, pork or prawns, salt and pepper. If using pork, crumble the raw pork in with fingers (see video). Mix through.

4. Heat 1/2 tbsp vegetable oil and drizzle of sesame oil in a non stick skillet over medium heat. Add a bit of garlic and quickly saute (10 seconds) and push into centre of skillet.

5. Ladle in 1/4 of batter. Use spatular to push edges in to form a round(ish) shape.

6. Cook until the underside is light golden (about 1 1/2 minutes) then flip and cook the other side for 1 minute. The raw meat will cook through in this time. Repeat with remaining egg to make 4 omelettes (use 2 pans if you can!).

7. Slide omelette onto plate. Pour over sauce. Sprinkle with sesame seeds and green onions, if using.

8. Serve with a side of rice and steamed vegetables of choice. Double the sauce if you want enough to pour over the rice and veggies!

Prep Time: 10 Minutes

Cook Time: 1hrs 15 Minutes

Servings: 5-6

Ingredients

Roasted Cauliflower:

- 1kg / 2 lb cauliflower florets (1 very large, 1 1/2 medium or 2 small cauliflower heads)
- 2 tbsp extra virgin olive oil
- 1/2 tsp sea salt
- 1/8 tsp pepper

Cheese Sauce (Mornay Sauce):

- 60g / 4 tbsp unsalted butter
- 3½ tbsp flour , plain / all-purpose
- 1 cup milk (full fat best)
- 1 cup cream (or more milk)
- 1/2 tsp cooking salt
- 1/4 tsp nutmeg powder (freshly grated is best)
- 1 cup Red Leicester cheese (or cheddar), grated

- 1/2 cup gruyère cheese, grated (or other melting cheese of choice)

Topping:

- 1/2 cup Red Leicester cheese (or cheddar), grated
- 1/2 cup gruyère cheese, grated (or other melting cheese of choice)

Instructions

Roasted Cauliflower:

1. Preheat oven to 220°C / 430°F (200°C fan).
2. Toss cauliflower in oil, salt and pepper. Spread on a large tray.
3. Roast 20 minutes (don't turn). Cauliflower should still be a bit firm, but with some colour on them. Remove from oven.
4. Turn oven down to 180°C/350°F.

Cheese Sauce (Mornay Sauce):

1. Heat milk: Heat milk and cream until hot – either on the stove or in microwave.

2. Make roux: Melt butter in a large saucepan or small pot over medium heat. Add flour and cook, stirring regularly, for 3 minutes.

3. Add milk: While stirring, pour in half the milk. Once the roux is dissolved into the milk (mixture will thicken), stir in remaining milk. Stir on the heat for 1 minute – mixture should be thick enough to coat a wooden spoon.

4. Add cheese: Turn the stove off, but leave the pot on the turned off stove. Stir in salt, nutmeg and both cheeses. The cheese will thicken the mixture so it's like a thick sauce.

5. Mix in cauliflower: Add cauliflower and toss to coat in the sauce.

Bake:

1. Fill baking dish: Transfer mixture to a 2L / 2qt baking dish (30 x 20 x 5cm / 12 x 8 x 2").

2. Top with cheese: Sprinkle over gruyère followed Red Leicester cheese.

3. Bake at 180°C/350°F for 30 minutes until the cheese is melted, and cauliflower is bubbly and golden.

4. Serve: Sprinkle with parsley if desired. Stand 5 minutes then serve!

Prep Time: 15 Minutes

Cook Time: 15 Minutes

Servings: 2

Ingredients

Bechamel:

- 1/2 cup milk
- 1/2 cup cream (pure or heavy / thickened)
- 1 1/2 tbsp / 25g unsalted butter
- 1 1/2 tbsp flour , plain / all-purpose
- 1/4 tsp cooking salt
- 1 pinch white pepper
- 1/8 tsp nutmeg, preferably freshly ground

Sandwich:

- 4 slices sourdough bread , 1.5cm / ⅗" thick
- 8 slices Swiss or gruyere cheese (165g / 6 oz, enough for 2 layers a sandwich)
- 120g / 4 oz ham slices, preferably smoked
- 4 tsp Dijon mustard
- 30g / 2 tbsp unsalted butter

Topping:

- 1/2 cup gruyere cheese, shredded (packed cup)
- 3 tbsp parmesan, finely shredded

Instructions

1. Preheat oven to 200°C/390°F (180°C fan).

Béchamel Sauce:

2. Heat milk and cream: Place milk and cream in a saucepan over medium heat. Heat until steaming, but don't let it boil. Set aside.
3. Make roux: Melt butter in a separate small saucepan over medium heat, then turn the heat down to low. Add flour and cook, stirring almost constantly, for 3 minutes. Don't let it brown.
4. Add hot milk: While stirring, add half the milk. Once incorporated into the roux, mix in remaining milk, nutmeg, salt and pepper.
5. Thicken: Mix for 30 seconds to a minute or until it thickens into a spreadable and soft butter-like consistency (ie. not runny). If you have lumps, whisk until gone. Remove from heat (it is OK if it cools).

Assemble For Pan Frying:

1. Spread with Bechamel: Spread half the béchamel over the 4 slices of bread, as though you are buttering them to make normal sandwiches! (Reserve half the béchamel for topping)

2. Cheese + Dijon: Top two pieces of bread with 2 slices of gruyere or Swiss cheese each (fold as needed to make them fit). Then spread the cheese with half the Dijon Mustard (this might sound weird, but see in post for why we do this!).

3. Ham + Dijon: Top with ham, then spread ham with remaining Dijon mustard.

4. Top each of the two slices with 2 more slices of cheese (again, folding as needed), then close sandwiches with the other slices.

Pan Fry:

1. Melt butter in a skillet over medium to medium-high heat. Place sandwiches in the skillet, and cook for 2 minutes, pressing down lightly with an egg flip or spatula, until a deep golden brown.

2. Turn and cook the other side until golden brown. Transfer to a baking tray.

Bake Then Broil:

1. Topping: Slather remaining béchamel thickly on the upper pieces of bread. Sprinkle with Gruyere, then parmesan.
2. Bake and broil: Bake 15 minutes, then switch to the grill/broiler for 3 minutes and grill until the top is golden and bubbling.

Serve:

1. Immediately transfer to warmed serving plates, with knives and fork for serving (it's too messy to eat with hands.) For a traditional French bistro experience, add a side of fries and leafy greens lightly dressed in French Dressing or a basic vinaigrette. Devour and weep with joy! (Over the sandwich that is, not the salad!)

Prep Time: 15 Minutes

Cook Time: 25 Minutes

Servings: 4-5

Ingredients

Cinnamon Pumpkin:

- 400g / 14 oz pumpkin or butternut squash (pre-peeled weight), peeled then sliced in 1cm / ½" thick slices then bite size wedges
- 2 tbsp extra virgin olive oil
- 1 tsp cinnamon
- 1/2 tsp all spice
- 1/4 tsp salt

SALAD:

- 800g/ 28oz canned lentils , well drained & patted dry
- 2 cups (packed) rocket/arugula leaves (preferably baby, otherwise hand-tear large ones)
- 1/2 red onion , finely sliced
- 3 tsp fresh thyme leaves

Honey Walnuts (Optional, Can Just Use Plain Walnuts,):

- 3/4 cup walnuts (or pecans)
- 1 1/2 tbsp honey (must be runny, so warm if super-thick), or maple syrup
- 1/4 tsp cinnamon
- Pinch of salt

Dressing:

- 2 tbsp red wine vinegar
- 2 tbsp honey
- 4 tbsp extra virgin olive oil
- 1 garlic clove (small), finely grated
- 1/4 tsp allspice powder
- 1/4 tsp ginger powder
- Salt and pepper

Instructions

Pan-Roasted Spiced Pumpkin:

2. Toss pumpkin with 1 tbsp olive oil, cinnamon, all spice and salt.

3. Pan roast: Heat a large non stick skillet with 1 tbsp olive oil over medium high heat. Add about half the pumpkin, spreading out into one layer. Cook for 3 minutes until golden. Turn and cook the other side for 3 minutes until golden and cooked through. Remove and let cool until just warm.

4. Repeat with other half of the pumpkin, adding a little more oil to the pan if required.

Honey Walnuts:

1. Toss: Place walnuts in a bowl, drizzle with honey, sprinkle with cinnamon and salt. Mix, spread on paper-lined baking tray.

2. Bake: Bake at 180°C/350°F (160°C fan) for 15 minutes, tossing once halfway. Leave to cool, then use fingers to roughly break walnuts up into slightly smaller pieces.

Salad:

1. Dressing: Place ingredients in a jar and shake well.

2. Toss: Place lentils, rocket, red onion, thyme and pumpkin in a large bowl. Pour over most of the Dressing, then gently toss.

3. Plate up: Pile up on serving platter. Sprinkle with candied walnuts. Drizzle over remaining Dressing, then serve!

Prep Time: 20 Minutes

Cook Time: 35 Minutes

Servings: 10-12

Ingredients

Quinoa:

- 1 cup quinoa , tri-colour (or other colour)
- 2 cups water

Salad:

- 1 cup cucumber, finely diced
- 1 carrot , medium, peeled and finely shredded
- 3 cups red cabbage , finely shredded (1/4 small or 1/8 large cabbage)
- 2 green onions , finely sliced
- 250g/ 8oz cherry tomatoes , small ones quartered, large ones cut into 6
- 1 cup shelled edamame , cooked per packet then cooled
- 1 red capsicum/bell pepper , finely chopped
- 1/2 cup coriander/cilantro leaves , finely chopped

Dressing:

- 5 tbsp soy sauce , light or all-purpose
- 2 tbsp mirin
- 2 tbsp rice wine vinegar (sub: cider, sherry or champagne vinegar)
- 2 tbsp sesame oil , toasted
- 2 1/2 tbsp canola, vegetable or grapeseed oil
- 2 1/2 tbsp Kewpie mayonnaise (sub whole-egg mayo such as Hellman's or S&W,)
- 2 1/2 tsp sugar (white or brown)
- 2 tsp ginger , freshly grated
- 1 garlic clove , crushed using garlic press or finely grated using microplane

Garnishes:

- 1/3 cup wasabi peas , crushed
- 1 tbsp sesame seeds , toasted

Instructions

Cook Quinoa:

1. Toast for extra flavour: Preheat oven to 200°C/390°F (180° fan) Spread quinoa on a tray. Bake 15 minutes,

stirring halfway, until it's lightly browned and smells nutty.

2. Rinse: Transfer to fine mesh sieve or strainer. Rinse under running water for 10 seconds, shake off excess water well.

3. Cook: Scrape into a medium saucepan. Add water, place lid on. Bring to simmer on medium heat, then lower stove to low and simmer for 15 minutes (or until all water is absorbed, tilt pot to check).

4. Rest: Remove from stove (lid still on) and rest for 10 minutes.

5. Fluff & cool: Remove lid, fluff quinoa with a fork and allow to fully cool before using. (Spread on a tray if you want to speed things up).

Salad:

1. Dressing: Place ingredients in a jar and shake well.

2. Toss salad! Place quinoa in a large bowl. Add all salad ingredients. Pour over dressing, toss very well.

3. Garnish: Either transfer to a large serving platter or individual bowls. Sprinkle generously with crushed Wasabi Peas and sesame seeds. Devour!

Prep Time: 15 Minutes

Cook Time: 15 Minutes

Servings: 8-10

Ingredients

Marinated Kale (Tenderised For Tastiness,):

- 5 kale stems (big and leafy, sub baby rocket/arugula but skip marinating)
- 1 tsp extra virgin olive oil
- Pinch of salt and pepper

Salad:

- 1 pomegranate , big, juicy (or 1 cup pomegranate arils,)
- 8 cups (120g/4.5oz) baby spinach (or baby rocket/arugula)
- 100g/3.5 oz blue cheese , crumbled yourself
- 1/2 cup dried cranberries (or raisins, craisins)

- 2 blood oranges , normal oranges, yellow peach, nectarine or grapefruit (optional, for extra colour/juicy/interest)

Honey Cinnamon Walnuts:

- 1 1/2 cup walnuts or pecans
- 1/4 cup honey (runny, so warm if super thick), or maple syrup
- 1/2 tsp cinnamon
- 1/8 tsp salt

Pomegranate Dressing:

- 2 tbsp pomegranate molasses
- 1 1/2 tbsp red wine vinegar (or white wine vinegar or cider vinegar)
- 4 tbsp extra virgin olive oil
- 1/2 tsp each salt and pepper

Instructions

Marinated Kale:

1. Remove leaves: Grab the base of the stalk then run your fist up the stalk to remove the leaves.

2. Slice: bundle the kale leaves on a chopping board, then slice 0.5 cm / 1/5" thick.

3. Scrunch: Place in bowl, drizzle with olive oil, sprinkle with salt and pepper. Use your hands to scrunch in order to soften leaves and coat everything with the oil. Do this for 20 seconds. Leave for 30 minutes to marinate – leaves will soften. Try it – much tastier than plain raw!

Honey Walnuts:

1. Toss: Place walnuts in a bowl, drizzle with honey, sprinkle with cinnamon and salt. Mix, spread on paper lined baking tray.

2. Bake: Bake at 180°C/350°F (160°C fan) for 15 minutes, tossing once halfway. Leave to cool, then use fingers to roughly break walnuts up into slightly smaller pieces.

Pomegranate Dressing:

1. Place ingredients in a jar and shake very well, being sure that there is no molasses left on the bottom of the jar. (Shake in jar is better than whisking to bring this dressing together).

Remove Pomegranate Seeds:

2. Cut pomegranate in half. Over a bowl, turn cut face downwards, then use a wooden spoon to (very!) firmly smack the back of the pomegranate. The seeds will fly out through your fingers into the bowl. It's very satisfying!!!

3. Keep smacking all over the skin until the seeds are all out. Pick out any white pith that fell out, then use seeds per recipe. You will probably get some juices pooling in the bowl; add this to the dressing too.

Slice Fruit (If Using):

1. Peaches, nectarines: Halve, remove stone, then cut into 4mm / 1/6" slices.

2. Grapefruit, oranges: Cut off peel and pith, then segment (see this video at 41 sec for demo)

Assemble:

1. Dress greens lightly: Place kale and spinach leaves in a giant bowl. Drizzle with about 3 tablespoons of Dressing then toss very well.

2. Layer half: Pour half kale/spinach into a large serving bowl. Sprinkle with 1/3 EACH of walnuts, blue cheese (crumbled), pomegranates, orange segments, and cranberries.

3. Presentation layer: Top with remaining kale & spinach, then remaining walnuts, blue cheese, pomegranates, orange segments and cranberries. Drizzle over remaining dressing just before serving.

4. Serving: Best served freshly assembled but this salad will hold up much better than most because kale doesn't go as soggy once dressing, it's even good the next day!

Prep Time: 10 Minutes

Cook Time: 15 Minutes

Servings: 2-4

Ingredients

Choose Pasta

- 200g / 7 oz short pasta like orecchiette penne, macaroni, spaghetti
- 160g/6 oz long pasta - spaghetti, fettucine

Garlic Butter Mushrooms For Pasta

- 400g / 14 oz mushrooms , sliced 1/2 cm / 1/5" thick
- 50g / 3 tbsp unsalted butter , separated
- 1 tbsp olive oil
- 2 garlic cloves, finely minced
- 1/2 tsp each salt and pepper
- 1/2 cup freshly grated parmesan cheese (or 1/4 cup store bought grated)

To Serve

- Parsley , finely chopped

- Parmesan cheese , grated

Instructions

Pasta

1. Bring a large pot of salted water to the boil. Add the pasta into the pot when you start cooking the mushrooms.
2. Cook pasta per packet instructions minus 1 minute. RESERVE 1 mugful of pasta cooking liquid, then drain pasta.

Mushrooms

1. Melt half butter and all oil in a large skillet over heat.
2. Add mushrooms and cook until water has leeched then evaporated, and the mushrooms start to turn golden around edges - around 5 minutes.
3. Halfway through cooking, add salt & pepper.
4. Add garlic and remaining butter, cook for 2 minutes until mushrooms and garlic are golden.
5. Add pasta, about 3/4 cup of reserved pasta water and parmesan. Toss gently or until water reduces and thickens into a saucy glaze that coats the pasta. If the pasta dries out, add more pasta water.

6. Taste and add more salt and pepper if needed.

7. Remove from stove and serve immediately, garnished with fresh parsley and parmesan cheese.

Prep Time: 10 Minutes

Cook Time: 20 Minutes

Servings: 6-8

Ingredients

Green Bean Salad:

- 500g / 1 lb green beans, ends trimmed, cut into 5cm / 2" pieces
- 3 tomatoes, cut into thin wedges
- 1 avocado (large, or 2 medium) diced into 1.5cm / 2/3" pieces
- 1/2 red capsicum / bell pepper, diced
- 1/2 red onion, finely diced

Creamy Avocado Dressing:

- 1/2 cup ripe avocado (smush into cup to measure, or estimate - 1/2 medium avo)
- 3 tbsp extra virgin olive oil
- 3 tbsp sour cream or yogurt (Greek or plain, unsweetened) - OPTIONAL
- 2 tbsp lemon juice

- 1 garlic clove, small, minced using garlic crusher
- 4 tbsp water (to thin out, it's very rich!)
- 1/2 tsp salt
- 1/4 tsp black pepper

Instructions

Dressing:

1. Place all ingredients into a Nutribullet or small food processor and blitz until smooth (including any Extra Flavouring Options suggested in the standalone Creamy Avocado Dressing recipe).
2. Use water to thin to just pourable consistency (so it's not super gloopy and thick). Taste and add the following to taste: salt, pepper, lemon, oil.

Salad:

1. Steam green beans using method of choice until soft (I microwave, 5 minutes on high). Drain then leave to cool and dry.
2. Place remaining salad ingredients in a large bowl with the beans. Drizzle with half the Dressing. Toss. Serve with remaining Dressing on the side.

3. It looks a bit of a mess once tossed. If you're serving to impress, just drizzle the Avocado Dressing over and take to the table like that

Prep Time: 15 Minutes

Cook Time: 1hrs 20 Minutes

Servings: 6-8

Ingredients

- 700g / 1.4lb potato , cut into 2cm / 4/5" pieces

Filling:

- 3 tbsp vegetable oil
- 1.5 tsp black mustard seeds
- 1 tsp cumin seeds
- 1 tsp fennel seeds
- 15 curry leaves, fresh
- 1 tbsp garlic, finely grated
- 1 onion, finely chopped (brown, white, yellow)
- 1/2 tsp turmeric powder
- 2 tsp curry powder
- 1/2 tsp chili powder, adjust spiciness to taste
- 1 tbsp tomato paste
- 1 tomato chopped into 1.5cm / 1/2" pieces
- 1 zucchini chopped into 1.5cm / 1/2" pieces

- 1 carrot chopped into 1.5cm / 1/2" pieces
- 1/2 cauliflower (small), cut/broken into small florets (3 cups)
- 1/2 tsp black pepper
- 1 tsp salt
- 2 cups water
- 1 cup frozen green peas

Puff Pastry Crust:

- 2 sheets puff pastry
- 1 egg, lightly whisked

Serving:

- Plain yogurt
- Coriander/cilantro leaves, option (decorative only, pictured)

Asterisk-Marked - Can Be Substituted with Any Vegetables That Can Be Cooked. Use 8 Cups Total.

Instructions

Mashed Potato:

1. Bring a pot of water to the boil then cook potato for 12 - 15 minutes until very soft.
2. Drain, mash and set aside.

Filling:

1. Sizzling spices: Heat oil in a dutch oven or pot over high heat. Add black mustard seeds, cumin and fennel seeds. Let them sizzle for 15 seconds - careful, they might pop!
2. Curry leaves: Then add curry leaves and stir for 15 seconds.
3. Aromatics: Add garlic, ginger and onion. Cook for 4 to 5 minutes until onion is tinged with gold.
4. Tomato: Add tomato paste and tomato, cook for 30 seconds.
5. Spices: Add curry powder, turmeric and chilli. Cook for 30 seconds.
6. Most Veg: Add zucchini, carrot and cauliflower. Stir well to coat in the spice paste.
7. Water: Add water, salt and pepper. Stir, bring to a simmer then put the lid on and reduce heat to medium low (so it's simmer gently).
8. Cook & reduce: Cook for 15 minutes until vegetables are soft. Then remove lid and simmer for 5 minutes to reduce liquid a bit.
9. Add mash: Remove from stove. Add peas and potato, mix through well.
10. Taste: Taste and add more salt and pepper if needed.

11. Cool: Place lid on and cool for at least 30 minutes (even overnight is fine).

Assembly & Baking:

1. Preheat oven to 180°C/350°F (all oven types).
2. Grease a large pie dish with butter, or oil spray Drape in a puff pastry sheet.
3. Fill with Filling - slightly mounded is fine.
4. Fold in the corners of the puff pastry sheet.
5. Top with puff pastry sheet - turn 90 degrees to the base puff pastry sheet .
6. Fold the overhang puff pastry under itself - no need to be neat here, this is a rustic pie!
7. Egg wash: Brush with egg, cut a 2cm / 1" cross in the middle (to let steam escape).
8. Bake 50 to 60 minutes, until the top is very deep golden and flaky.
9. Stand 5 minutes then slice to serve. A dollop of plain yogurt goes well with this!

20. Roasted Eggplant Lentil Salad

Prep Time: 15 Minutes

Cook Time: 5hrs 20 Minutes

Servings: 4-8

Ingredients

Tasty Lentils!

- 1 cup dried green or brown lentils (or French/puy) for canned)
- 1 cup vegetable or chicken broth (or water + 1 bouillon cube, crumbled)
- 1 1/2 cups water
- 1 large garlic clove, smashed, skin removed
- Lemon peel (about 1.5 x 5 cm / 3/4 x 2")
- 1 bay leaf, dry or fresh
- 2 sprigs thyme, or 1/2 tsp dried thyme
- 1 rib celery, broken into 3 or 4 pieces (or just a handful of celery leaves, can skip)

Roasted Eggplant:

- 700g / 1.4 lb eggplant / aborigine (2 medium)
- 2 1/2 tbsp olive oil

- 1/4 tsp EACH salt and pepper

Garlic Lemon Dressing:

- 2 tbsp lemon juice (or cider vinegar, white or red wine vinegar)
- 4 tbsp extra virgin olive oil
- 1 tsp Dijon mustard
- 1 garlic clove, minced using garlic press
- 1 tsp thyme leaves, fresh (or 1/2 ts dried - can omit, or other herbs)
- 1 tsp sugar, optional
- 1/2 tsp EACH salt + black pepper

Salad:

- 250g/ 8 oz cherry tomatoes, halved (large quartered)
- 2 handfuls rocket / arugula lettuce, torn into 5cm/2" pieces
- 60g/ 2 oz feta, crumbled (or more!)

Instructions

Dressing - shake in a jar.

Lentils:

1. Place Lentil ingredients in a saucepan, bring to simmer over medium heat. Place lid on then lower heat to medium low so it's simmering gently.

2. Cook for 20 minutes (for al dente, my preference), or 25 minutes (for soft), stirring occasionally.

3. Drain, then pick out all the flavouring bits (garlic etc). BRIEFLY rinse to get grit off - don't wash off all the flavour! Shake off excess water well.

Roasted Eggplant:

1. Preheat oven to 240°C / 450°F (220°C fan). Line a tray with parchment/baking paper.

2. Cut eggplant into large cubes - 3 cm / 1.2". Place in large bowl, drizzle with oil, salt and pepper.

3. Toss well, then immediately spread on tray and roast 20 minutes. Flip, then roast for a further 10 minutes - edges should be caramelised, soft inside, but they're not shrivelled up and dismal.

Assemble:

1. Add tomato and rocket into lentils, drizzle over most of the Dressing then toss.

2. Pour onto serving platter. Pile over eggplant.

3. Drizzle eggplant with remaining Dressing, sprinkle with feta . Serve warm or at room temp! Great with a side of flatbread or this easy crusty bread.

21. Homemade Heinz Baked Beans

Prep Time: 5 Minutes

Cook Time: 30 Minutes

Servings: 8-10

Ingredients

Beans – Choose One:

- 2 cups (14 oz) dried Navy beans (aka Haricot) or other white beans
- 3 x 400g/14oz cans haricot/navy beans, cannellini or any white beans, drained

Baked Beans:

- 2 cups chicken stock/broth, low sodium, OR homemade vegetable stock
- 1 cup water
- 2 tsp Worcestershire sauce
- 6 tbsp ketchup or Aussie/British tomato sauce
- 2 tbsp tomato paste
- 3 tbsp brown sugar

- 1 tbsp apple cider vinegar
- 1/2 tsp garlic powder (or more onion powder)
- 1/2 tsp onion powder (or more garlic powder)
- 1/2 tsp black pepper
- 1 tsp salt

Sauce Thickening:

- 8 tsp corn flour / cornstarch
- 1/4 cup water

Instructions

Cook Dried Beans:

1. No need to do these steps if using canned beans, start with Step 1 under "Baked Beans" below.
2. Soak beans in a big bowl of water for 8 – 24 hrs, then drain.
3. Skim foam – Place beans in a large pot of water over high heat. Bring to a simmer, then skim off foam.
4. Simmer Reduce heat so it's simmering gently (medium or medium low). Partially cover with lid (leaving a crack for steam to escape), then cook for 1 – 1.5 hrs until just tender. (Start checking at 45 min).

Beans should be still slightly firm on inside (they're cooked more in the sauce). Drain, use per recipe.

Baked Beans:

1. Mix – Place all Baked Beans ingredients in a pot (except beans) and stir, then add beans.
2. Simmer – Bring to a simmer, then lower heat to medium low and simmer for 20 minutes, without the lid. Stir every now and then so the beans don't catch on the bottom of the pot.

Thicken Sauce:

1. Mix cornflour with water. Pour into pot while stirring, then cook for 2 minutes until sauce thickens – it will thicken quickly.
2. Check for salt: Taste and add more salt if needed.
3. Serve it the traditional way – piled over hot buttered toast. Or ladle into bowls, eat with a spoon and dunk in hot crusty bread! Popular breads – simple crusty Artisan bread, Irish Soda Bread (No yeast) and No Yeast Sandwich Bread

Prep Time: 10 Minutes

Cook Time: 20 Minutes

Servings: 8-9

Ingredients

- 1/4 cup flour , plain / all purpose
- 1/4 cup cornflour / cornstarch
- 1/4 tsp baking soda (or 3/4 tsp baking powder)
- 1 egg
- 2 tbsp milk (any type)
- 2 cups fresh corn kernels, raw (2 cobs) (canned or frozen also fine)
- 1/2 cup parmesan, finely grated
- 3/4 cup green onions, sliced
- 1/2 cup coriander/cilantro, roughly chopped (sub more green onion)

For Cooking:

- 1/2 cup vegetable oil
- Oil spray

Serving - Choose:

- Avocado sauce
- Sour cream, ketchup (don't judge until you've tried it!)

Instructions

1. Preheat oven to 120°C / 250°F and set a wire rack on a baking tray.
2. Place flour, cornflour and baking soda in a bowl, mix to combine.
3. Add egg and milk, mix until incorporated (batter will be lumpy and thick).
4. Add corn, parmesan, green onions and coriander. Mix until all the corn is evenly coated in batter.
5. Add enough oil into the skillet so it just covers the base. Heat over medium high heat.
6. Spray the underside of a spatula with oil (so batter won't stick when you flatten).
7. Place 1/4 cup batter into skillet (ice cream scooper with lever is handy), then flatten to 1cm thick. Repeat with 2 or 3 more, but don't crowd the skillet.
8. Cook 3 minutes until deep golden and crisp, then flip and cook the other side for 2 – 3 minutes.

9. Transfer to rack and keep warm in oven. Repeat with remaining fritters, using more oil as necessary.

10. Serve with sauce of choice for dunking!

Prep Time: 30 Minutes

Cook Time: 10 Minutes

Servings: 5

Ingredients

- 500g / 1 lb hot smoked salmon, store bought, any flavor

Quick Pickled Onion:

- 1 small red onion, halved then finely sliced
- 1 cup (250 ml) apple cider vinegar (enough to just cover onion), sub white wine vinegar
- 1 tsp salt
- 2 tsp white sugar

Yoghurt Ranch Dressing:

- 2 cups Greek yoghurt, full fat recommended
- 3 tbsp extra virgin olive oil
- 1 garlic clove , minced
- 1/4 cup fresh chives, finely chopped
- 1/4 cup fresh dill, finely chopped

- 1/2 tsp EACH onion powder, garlic powder, salt, black pepper
- 1 1/2 tsp white sugar
- 3 tbsp lemon juice

Marinated Kale:

- 4 cups (packed) kale , torn into bite size pieces
- 2 tsp extra virgin olive oil
- Pinch of salt

Salad:

- 2 pieces fruit - nectarines, peaches, grapefruit or blood oranges (get whatever's ripe and juicy, or sub normal oranges)
- 10 cups cos lettuce / romaine torn or cut into bite size pieces
- 1 small fennel , shaved (0.5 mm / 1/5" thickness) or finely sliced
- 1 handful snow pea sprouts (can omit)
- 3/4 cup (75g) parmesan , shredded

Instructions

1. Flake salmon: Use two forks to flake salmon into large chunks.

2. Dressing: Mix the Yoghurt Ranch Dressing ingredients in a bowl. Adjust olive oil + lemon juice to taste. Leave 20 minutes.

3. Pickle Onions: Place ingredients in a bowl, toss to coat. Set aside for 1 hour+ or until onion is softened (if in a rush, make sure the onion is finely sliced = faster pickle). Drain.

4. Marinated Kale: Place kale in a large bowl, drizzle with oil then sprinkle with salt. Use your fingers to massage the oil onto the leaves - you want to ensure every part of the kale is coated in oil. Set aside for 30 minutes or until kale is softened.

Slice Fruit:

1. Nectarines/peaches option- halve then finely slice.

2. Grapefruit/blood orange option - segment per . Squeeze all remaining juice out of the membrane after segmenting, mix into dressing.

Assemble:

1. Place lettuce, kale, fennel, 1/2 cup onion in bowl. Drizzle with about 1 cup dressing and 1/3 cup

parmesan. Toss well to coat. Taste, add more parmesan or salt if you want, or more dressing.

2. Pile half dressed lettuce onto serving platter. Flake over half the salmon and half the fruit. Scatter with more red onion.

3. Top with remaining lettuce, salmon, fruit and onion (might not use all onion).

4. Drizzle with some dressing (might not use all, serve remainder on side). Scatter over snow pea sprouts, sprinkle with remaining parmesan. Place on table and let everyone help themselves!

Prep Time: 15 Minutes

Cook Time: 50 Minutes

Servings: 10-14

Ingredients

- 8 heaped cups plain white bread, crust on, cut into 2.5cm / 1 "cubes (600g/1.2lb)
- 500g/ 1 lb pork sausages, good quality
- 50g/ 3 tbsp butter, unsalted
- 1/2 onion, finely diced
- 1 large celery stalk, sliced 3mm / 1/8" thick
- 1 granny smith apple, skin left on, diced into 0.5 cm / 1/5" cubes
- 1/3 cup pecans, roughly chopped
- 1 cup (250 ml) chicken stock/broth, low sodium
- 1/3 cup (85 ml) cream, heavy / thickened (low fat also ok)
- 1 tbsp fresh sage, finely chopped
- 1 tsp fresh thyme leaves
- 1/4 tsp each salt and pepper

Garnishes (Optional)

- 30g / 2 tbsp butter, melted (extra for brushing)
- Thyme leaves, small sage leaves, chopped parsley, optional garnish

Instructions

1. Preheat oven to 160°C/320°F.
2. Spread bread out on tray (squished is fine). Bake for 8 minutes until lightly toasted – pale gold ok, should be soft on inside but crispy on outside. Transfer into large bowl.
3. Meanwhile, place about 1 tsp butter in a large skillet over high heat. Once melted, add sausage and cook, breaking it up as you go.
4. Once cooked with a few golden bits, pour over bread (yes, including all the fat!).
5. Return skillet to stove, turn down to medium. Add remaining butter. Once melted, add onion, cook 2 minutes.
6. Add celery and apple, cook for 3 minutes.
7. Add pecans, chicken stock, creamy, sage, thyme, salt and pepper. Stir.

8. Bring to simmer, then cook for 2 minutes, then pour it into the bowl. Mix well, ensuring all the bread is evenly coated. Get in there with your hands if needed!

9. Taste and add more salt if needed (depends on saltiness of sausage).

10. Transfer into a 2 litre / 2 quarts baking dish. Cover with foil, bake 40 minutes.

11. Remove foil, brush with Extra melted butter if desired. Then broil/grill on high for 2 to 4 minutes until the top is nicely browned (watch it carefully - but be brave! Colour = flavour!).

12. Serve warm, sprinkled with parsley, fresh thyme or some small fresh sage leaves if desired!

Prep Time: 20 Minutes

Cook Time: 2hrs 10 Minutes

Servings: 10

Ingredients

Sweet Potato Mash:

- 1.75kg / 3.5lb sweet potato (3 large or 6 smaller ones)
- 1/2 cup (115g) sour cream
- 1/2 cup (50g) parmesan, freshly grated
- 2 garlic cloves, finely minced
- 3/4 tsp salt
- 1/4 tsp black pepper

Browned Butter & Crispy Sage:

- 250g / 8oz butter, salted, cut into 2cm/1" cubes
- 15 sage leaves
- TOPPING:
- 3/4 cup panko breadcrumbs
- 1/2 cup (50g) parmesan , finely grated
- 1/4 tsp each salt and pepper

- 150g / 5oz bacon, streaky, cooked until golden then finely chopped

Instructions

Bake & Mash:

1. Preheat oven to 180°C/350°F.
2. Place potatoes on a foil lined tray. Bake for 1 hour 15 minutes (small) to 1 hour 40 minutes (large) until knife can be easily inserted into the centre.
3. Cool potatoes until they can be handled (but still piping hot inside!) or use tea towel to handle.

Browned Butter & Crispy Sage:

1. Meanwhile, place butter in a large silver saucepan over medium heat.
2. Once melted and starts to foam, add sage leaves. Cook 1 minute or until golden brown, then fish through the foam to find the leaves and drain on paper towels (will crisp when cool).
3. Continue to leave butter on stove until foam dies down and you see black bits on the bottom of the pan (it will smell nutty).

4. Strain through paper towel lined sieve - should have 180ml or so.

TOPPING:

1. Crumble sage leaves in your hand (chop if not fully crisp) and place in bowl.
2. Add 1/4 cup Browned Butter, panko, parmesan, garlic, salt and pepper, mix.

Mash:

1. Cut slits down the middle of the potatoes then scoop flesh out into a bowl.
2. Add 1/4 cup Browned Butter (below), sour cream, parmesan, salt and pepper. Mash or use electric beater to mash until smooth (if using food processor, be careful not to overdo as it will make potato gluey).

Assemble & Bake:

1. Place half the potato in a baking dish (2 litre / 2 quarts). Make swirls across surface with spoon (as catchment for butter!), then drizzle over 1/4 cup Browned Butter. Cover the butter pools with remaining potato - the less you disturb the butter, the better!

2. Sprinkle over Topping. Bake 25 minutes until top is golden brown and edges are bubbling.

3. Sprinkle with crumbled bacon, then bake a further 5 minutes. If you've got any leftover butter, drizzle it on then serve!

Prep Time: 30 Minutes

Cook Time: 45 Minutes

Servings: 5

Ingredients

Cannelloni Sauce:

- 1 tbsp olive oil
- 2 garlic cloves, minced
- 1/2 onion, finely chopped
- 1 carrot, small, finely chopped (optional)
- 1 celery rib, finely chopped (optional)
- 800g / 28oz crushed tomato, canned
- 2 cups (500ml) chicken stock / broth, low sodium (or vegetable)
- 1/2 tsp EACH thyme, oregano, salt, pepper
- 1/4 tsp chili flakes, optional

Spinach Beef Filling:

- 1 tbsp olive oil
- 2 garlic cloves , minced
- 1/2 onion , finely chopped

- 500g / 1lb beef mince, lean
- 250g / 8oz frozen spinach, chopped, thawed, excess liquid squeezed out
- 1 beef bouillon cube, crumbled
- 1/2 tsp pepper
- 1 tsp Worcestershire Sauce

Cannelloni:

1. 21 - 24 cannelloni tubes (220g/7oz) OR 10 Manicotti tubes
2. 2 cups mozzarella cheese , freshly grated (or other melting cheese)
3. Chopped parsley , garnish (optional)

Instructions

Cannelloni Sauce:

1. Heat oil in a large saucepan or pot over medium high heat. Add garlic and onion, cook 2 minutes. Add carrot and celery, cook 5 minutes.
2. Add remaining Sauce ingredients then stir. Bring to simmer lower heat to medium, cover with lid and simmer for 10 minutes.

3. Use a stick blender to blitz until smooth (or cool slightly and use blender or food processor). Set aside.

Spinach Beef Filling:

1. Heat oil in a large skillet over high heat. Add onion and garlic, cook 2 minutes.
2. Add beef and cook, breaking it up as you go, until it all changes from red to brown.
3. Stir in spinach, then add crumbled beef cube, Worcestershire sauce, pepper and 1 cup of Cannelloni Sauce. Stir, cook 2 minutes.
4. Remove and cool slightly.

Assembly And Baking:

1. Preheat oven to 180°C/350°F.
2. Transfer Beef Filling into a piping bag with a wide nozzle. Stand cannelloni tubes upright in a container, then pipe filling in. (Or do this step with teaspoon/finger/dinner knife!).
3. Spread about 1 1/4 cups Sauce in a 23x33cm / 9x13" dish. Lay the cannelloni on top, then pour over remaining Sauce.
4. Sprinkle with cheese, loosely cover with foil.

5. Bake 25 minutes, remove foil then bake a further 10 minutes until the cheese is bubbly with some golden spots.

6. Remove from oven, sprinkle with parsley if using then serve!

Prep Time: 10 Minutes

Cook Time: 5 Minutes

Servings: 4

Ingredients

Sauce:

- 2 1/2 tbsp soy sauce
- 3 tbsp honey
- 1 1/2 tbsp Oyster sauce
- 1 1/2 tbsp Chinese cooking wine, Mirin or dry sherry
- 2 tbsp water
- 1 tsp coarsely crushed black pepper (or 1/2 tsp normal ground black pepper)

Stir Fry

- 2 tbsp peanut oil (or vegetable or canola oil)
- 1 garlic clove , finely minced
- 1/2 onion , peeled and sliced
- 500g/1 lb thinly sliced tenderloin, flank, sirloin/Porterhouse/strip, or any other cut of steak suitable for stir frying (Notes 3)

Instructions

1. Mix the Sauce ingredients in a bowl.

2. Heat the oil in a wok or large heavy based skillet over high heat until it is smoking.

3. Add the onion and garlic and cook for 1 minute or until the onion becomes translucent. Keep it moving so the garlic doesn't burn.

4. Add the beef and stir fry for 1 minute until just cooked to your liking, then remove into bowl.

5. Turn the heat down to medium high, pour in Sauce - it will start simmering very quickly! Let it cook for 1 minute or so until it becomes syrupy - the bubbles will be larger and caramel colour.

6. Add the beef and onion back into the wok, along with any juices pooled on the plate. Toss in the sauce until just warmed through - 1 minute at most. Don't overcook the beef - that would be tragic!

7. Serve immediately with rice - or for a low carb, low cal option, try Cauliflower Rice!

Prep Time: 10 Minutes

Cook Time: 5 Minutes

Servings: 4

Ingredients

Sweet Potato:

- 1kg / 2 lb sweet potato cut into 2cm / 4/5" cubes
- 2 tbsp olive oil
- 1/2 tsp salt and pepper
- SALAD:
- 200g/ 7oz baby spinach (or rocket/arugula)
- 1/2 red onion, finely sliced
- 3/4 cup sliced almond, toasted
- 90g/ 3oz feta, crumbled
- 3/4 cup dried cranberries
- 2 cups cooked wild rice, warm

Honey Lemon Mustard Dressing:

- 3 tbsp lemon juice
- 5 tbsp extra olive oil
- 1.5 tbsp honey

- 2 tsp Dijon mustard
- 1 garlic clove, small, minced
- 1/2 tsp salt
- 1/2 tsp pepper

Instructions

1. Preheat oven to 200°C / 390°F.
2. Shake Dressing ingredients in a jar.
3. Toss sweet potato with olive oil, salt and pepper, spread onto tray.
4. Roast for 20 minutes, flip, then roast for a further 5 minutes until golden on edges.
5. Place baby spinach, onion and half almonds in a bowl. Drizzle with 2 tbsp Dressing, toss.
6. Drizzle warm rice with 1 tbsp Dressing, toss.
7. Spread spinach on serving platter. Top with rice, then sweet potato and cranberries.
8. Drizzle with remaining Dressing, then top with feta and remaining almonds. Serve!

Prep Time: 5Minutes

Cook Time: 10 Minutes

Servings: 4

Ingredients

Chicken Marinade:

- 600-750g / 1.2 - 1.5 lb chicken breasts (4 pieces) or boneless thigh
- Zest of 1 lime (zest before juicing)
- 4 tbsp lime juice (1 - 2 limes)
- 2 garlic cloves, minced
- 3 tbsp brown sugar
- 1/4 tsp pepper
- 1 tbsp olive oil
- 2 tbsp finely chopped cilantro/coriander (optional)
- 1 tbsp fish sauce (OR 2 tbsp soy sauce)

To Cook

- 1 - 2 tbsp olive oil

Instructions

1. Use fist (or rolling pin!) to pound fat end of chicken breast to about 1.7 cm / 2/3" thickness (not required for thigh).
2. Place chicken and Marinade in a ziplock bag, massage to distribute marinade evenly. Place on a plate or bowl and refrigerate for 24 hours (min 12 hrs, max 48 hrs - Note 3)
3. Remove chicken, discard Marinade. Cook using one method below.

To Cook (Cooked Internal Temp 165f/75c)

Stove:

1. Heat oil in a large skillet over medium high heat. Cook chicken for 3 minutes on each side or until caramelised and golden brown (see video!).

BBQ:

2. Brush grills with oil and heat to medium high (or medium if your BBQ is strong). Cook chicken for 3 minutes on each side until caramelised (see video!).
3. OVEN: Preheat oven to 425F/220C. Bake 15 minutes, then flick broiler/grill on high and grill for 3 minutes to caramelise surface & finish cooking.

Rest And Serve:

1. Transfer chicken to a serving plate, cover loosely with foil and rest for 3 minutes.
2. Garnish with extra coriander/cilantro, lime wedges and chilli if desired, then serve!

Prep Time: 20 Minutes

Cook Time: 5 Minutes

Servings: 8-10

Ingredients

Salad:

- 180g / 6 oz baby spinach
- 1 red onion (small), halved and finely sliced
- 375g / 12 oz ripe strawberries, sliced
- 2 avocados, quartered and sliced
- 120g / 4oz feta, crumbled

Candied Pecans:

- 1 tbsp (15g) butter, unsalted
- 3 tbsp white sugar
- 1 cup pecans, roughly chopped

Poppyseed Dressing:

- 1 tbsp eschallots (French onion), very finely chopped
- 2.5 tbsp white wine vinegar
- 5 tbsp olive oil

- 1.5 tbsp mayonnaise
- 1 tbsp white sugar
- 1 tbsp poppyseeds
- 3/4 tsp salt
- 1/4 tsp black pepper

Instructions

1. Place Dressing ingredients in a jar and shake well. Set aside for 10 minutes+ (keeps for a week).

Candied Pecans:

2. Place butter and sugar in a non stick skillet over medium high. When butter is melted, add nuts.
3. Stir 5 minutes - sugar will go sandy, then eventually melt into a caramel.
4. Once sugar melts, cook for 2 minutes then spread pecans out on tray.
5. Cool then break to separate.

Assemble Salad:

1. Place spinach and onion in a bowl, drizzle with about 3 tbsp Dressing, toss.

2. Transfer 1/3 spinach in a bowl. Scatter over 1/3 of each strawberries, avocado, feta, pecans. Drizzle with a bit of dressing.

3. Top with another 1/3 spinach, strawberries, avocado, feta, pecans, then a bit more Dressing. Repeat once more.

4. Serve immediately!